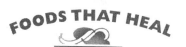

FOODS THAT HEAL

MAUREEN KENNEDY SALAMAN

S0-BYO-596

UNMASKING AND CONQUERING Depression

Practical, Natural Ways

to Break Its Grip

Without Using Drugs

STATFORD
PUBLISHING

IMPORTANT NOTICE

This book is neither a medical guide nor a manual for self-treatment. It is instead intended as a reference work only. The information in this book is meant to help you make informed choices about your health, but is not intended as a substitute for any treatment that may be prescribed or recommended by your doctor or health care practitioner. If you should suspect that you suffer from a medical condition or problem, you should seek competent medical care without delay

Unmasking and Overcoming Depression

Copyright © 2006
Maureen Kennedy Salaman
All rights reserved. No part of this book may be reproduced in any form or by any means without written consent of publisher/author.
ISBN 0-913087-30-0
First Printing

MKS, Inc.
1259 El Camino Real, Suite 1500
Menlo Park, California 94025
www.mksalaman.com
(650) 854-3922 telephone
(650) 854-5779 facsimile

Distributed by:
Maximum Living, Inc.
20071 Soulsbyville Road
Soulsbyville, California 95372-9748
www.maximizeyourlife.com
(209) 536-9300 telephone
(800) 445-4325 toll-free
(209) 536-9375 facsimile

Interior and cover design by:
Koechel Peterson & Associates, Inc., Minneapolis, MN

Cover photo by Russ Fischella

Printed in the United States of America

CONTENTS

———— ∞∞∞ ————

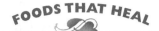

CHAPTER ONE

IT'S *NOT* ALL IN YOUR HEAD

*In the midst of winter,
I finally learned that there
was in me an invincible summer.*

—Albert Camus

LITTLE BILLY PARKER loves baseball. His favorite team is the San Francisco Giants. Billy is nine years old and lives in California with his mother near the Stanford Medical Center, where he goes for physical therapy for his cerebral palsy.

One day Billy and his mother were in the waiting room at Stanford, waiting for the nurse to call them.

"Mom," he began, his pale blue eyes gazing into hers with all the seriousness of an adult. "I want to be a professional baseball player."

Her heart was touched. She knew he meant it, and tears of sad disappointment welled up in her eyes. She wanted him to have whatever he desired, but this was too much. "Honey," she said, her voice catching, "you can't play baseball. Your little legs can't run fast."

Little Billy responded, "I wouldn't need to run fast. When I play baseball, I'll just hit them out of the park. Then I'll be able to walk."

I have no doubt that if Billy wants to play professional baseball, he will. Billy knows what some of us are still realizing: whatever handicap we are dealt with, whether it be cerebral palsy or depression, we are the best people to judge how we handle it, and what we want to do about it. Hope springs eternal, and there is always hope.

DEPRESSION CAUSED BY SEROTONIN SIGNALS

The first thing to realize about depression is that it is *not* all in your head. It can be caused by chemical imbalances that can be righted. Like Billy's cerebral palsy, it is not *the* reason to give up; it is *a* reason to try harder.

Post-traumatic stress disorder, clinical depression, and even stress are catchall words used by conventional medicine to conveniently box symptoms into a category so they can be diagnosed and treated with drugs. If you have been diagnosed with one of these "afflictions," don't let the pronouncement make you lose hope.

Depression is caused by reduced levels of serotonin, a brain chemical, or neurotransmitter, which influences hunger, aggression, sleep, and response to fear. Low serotonin levels act on the brain—the portion called the *amygdala*—which results in an inability to feel pleasure and enjoy life. Remember that depression can be temporary and is based on your body, not your brain. You always have the power to heal.

Traumatic events, environmental chemicals, pharmaceutical drugs, hormone fluctuations, viruses, and chemical addictions depress the body's levels of serotonin. These are temporary conditions that, when identified, can help turn the corner and let you into the light of happiness.

Here are some symptoms of low serotonin levels:

1. You awake every morning at about the same time and can't get back to sleep. Serotonin, you see, controls the sleep cycle.

2. You have no energy. You go to bed early and take naps during the day, but you are always dead tired.

3. You have trouble concentrating, forgetting why you went to the store and even where you are going. You lose items, then find them in odd places such as the refrigerator.

4. You lose interest in socializing and eventually stop answering the phone or the door.

5. As tired as your body is, your mind never seems to stop. Your body moves like a carted horse, but your mind races like an Indy 500 car. Your mind seems to turn against you, relentlessly reaching into the depths of your past bad experiences.

6. Hopelessness and disappointment threaten to overwhelm you.

MOVING BEYOND EMOTIONS FOR ANSWERS

Here are some causes of depression and fatigue that, once identified, can be a good start toward becoming healthy—and happy—again.

Nutritional Deficiencies

People who are deficient in thiamine (vitamin B1) and vitamin B6 are more prone to depression. The most promising nutrients to date for overcoming depression and fatigue are vitamins B3, B6, B12, and folic acid, amino acids, zinc, and magnesium, and essential fatty acids (EFAs). The B vitamins are essential for a healthy nervous system. About one third of the psychiatric population have low blood levels of B6 and zinc.

Food Allergies

Food allergies are so detrimental to the body that they cause nutritional deficiencies. An intolerance to gluten—a complex protein found in wheat, rye, barley, and oats—causes celiac disease, the destruction of the intestinal lining that in turn causes deficiencies of B vitamins.

Chemical Sensitivities

Have you heard of sick building syndrome? One of the symptoms is fatigue, and it is caused by an allergic reaction to the plethora of chemicals found in building materials, especially new buildings. When I get a new carpet, I spray it with a combination of hydrogen peroxide and water. Hyperactivity, mood swings, depression, and anxiety are all symptoms of chemical sensitivity.

Medications

Long-term use of certain pharmaceutical medications, such as some drugs used to control high blood pressure, sleeping pills, or, occasionally, birth control pills, can cause depression, as they steal invaluable B vitamins, such as folic acid, from your body. Even antidepressants and drugs prescribed for bipolar disorders can cause severe depression if taken inappropriately or in excess.

Illnesses

Having an underactive thyroid (hypothyroidism), even mildly, can cause depression. Up to 20 percent of all chronic depression cases may be caused by low thyroid hormones. A University of North Carolina study found that among women with mildly decreased thyroid function, the rate of those who had suffered depression at least once in their lives was almost three times as great as among those with normal thyroid function.

The Borna virus may be the cause of some cases of serious depression. The virus was first identified in the late 1800s among horses near the town of Borna, Germany. The horses stopped eating, walked in circles, and got sick. Some even killed themselves. Autopsies led scientists to the virus in the region of the horses' brains that controls emotions. Researchers have found a similar strain in humans.

Hormones

Women may experience depression twice as much as men, but men also lose hormones as they get older—some call it male menopause, or andro-pause. A lack of testosterone is associated with depression.

Alcohol, Nicotine, and Drug Abuse

Some people with depression use alcohol, nicotine, and mood-altering drugs as a way to ease its symptoms. But the use of these substances can also cause depression.

GETTING BACK ON TRACK

For every cause there is a solution. If you are convinced that you, or someone you know, cannot simply think your way to happiness, know that much can be done and learned to get you and your loved one back on track to a normal, happy, *joyous* life.

In the following chapters I will discuss these different reasons for depression and fatigue, how supplemental nutrition can help, and how the very drugs you are taking to ameliorate your prob-lems can be entrenching them and distorting your perspective on life.

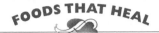
CHAPTER TWO

DEPRESSION AND HORMONES

> *If depression is creeping up and must be faced, learn something about the nature of the beast: you may escape without a mauling.*

—R. W. Shepherd

DAVID CREDITED THE PAIN of his divorce for his inability to sleep and the black mood he couldn't shake. It was understandable and natural, after all. He was nearing 50, living alone, and forced to ask permission to see his kids. While he considered the ten years he was married hell on earth, finding himself alone was no picnic either.

But something else was contributing to David's problem, and he didn't realize it; something that was causing his bad mood, unrelated to his divorce and the stress he was under.

MALE MENOPAUSE AND DEPRESSION

David was going through male menopause, or

andropause, a condition largely unrecognized and undiagnosed. It occurs as the male body loses testosterone over time. The production of testosterone increases rapidly at the start of puberty. Once men reach middle age, however, testosterone levels begin to drop by about one percent each year.

When getting tested for testosterone levels, make sure the test includes a measurement of "free" testosterone, not just "total." Only free hormones affect the body. For decades, men were only tested for total testosterone. Once they began testing for the free version, they were shocked. Researchers discovered that levels of free testosterone decline by as much as 40 percent between the ages of 40 and 70. Studies of men in combat show that severe stress and fear strongly lower testosterone.

Men who suffer from depression have lower levels of free testosterone than normal subjects. There are two reasons for this. The first is the brain. Certain regions of the brain, regions that influence mood and behavior, need testosterone to function properly.

A common sign of low testosterone is a change in mood and behavior. You find it easy to get angry at trivial incidents. Things you used to enjoy now seem like chores. Hope is elusive. Some researchers think that low testosterone levels are one reason why some men become grumpy, nervous, and irritable as they age.

The other reason low testosterone levels cause depression is because as testosterone levels drop, cortisol levels rise. (By the way, men also produce estrogen, although in much smaller amounts than women.) Cortisol is a hormone that the body produces in response to stress, anger, or fear. Too much cortisol can cause emotional overreaction—paranoia, misunderstanding, irrational fear, and depression. Do you feel more irritable in the morning? In normal people the level of cortisol in the bloodstream peaks in the morning, then decreases as the day progresses. In depressed people, however, cortisol peaks earlier in the morning and does not level off or decrease in the afternoon or evening.

As I researched the subject of andropause, I noticed that conventional medicine is recommending hormone replacement therapy for men using synthetic forms of testosterone. Do not make the same mistake women have been making for years. There are too many risks to ingesting synthetic anything, including the synthetic chemicals found in processed food. There are supplements and foods that can help raise testosterone, reduce cortisol, and alleviate "Grumpy Grandpa Syndrome."

ESTROGEN, TESTOSTERONE, AND DEPRESSION IN WOMEN

Much more is known about the affect of hormones on the mental well-being of women.

Kathy Bates' mood-swinging character in the movie *Fried Green Tomatoes* tore down walls and built them back up again while Jessica Tandy exhorted her to "take those hormones!" and get on with her life.

What men, women, and depression have in common are the adrenal glands. As people age, the adrenals make less hormones. In men—and women—testosterone is reduced, and in women, estrogen production slows to a crawl. A woman's ovaries produce estrogen as well as small amounts of testosterone.

Despite the fact that only a small amount is produced, testosterone helps women maintain muscle and bone strength. After menopause, testosterone levels drop. Estrogen replacement therapy can also reduce testosterone levels. While there are no standardized, agreed upon thresholds for what is "normal" testosterone levels for women, researchers find that low levels do affect them. Symptoms of low testosterone include low sex drive and desire, depression, loss of bone mass, low energy, moodiness, weakness, and muscle loss.

Low testosterone is called *hypogonadism.* Since testosterone is produced in daily cycles, levels vary by time of day, stage of menstruation/ menopause, and age. Some pharmaceutical drugs directly lower testosterone, such as Megace, ganciclovir, Nizoral, and some birth control pills.

The bottom line is that reduced and fluctuating levels of sex hormones in women and men contribute to depression, no matter what researchers and physicians choose to call it— menopause, postpartum depression, clinical depression, or premenstrual syndrome. And what they often don't tell you is you can help yourself naturally, without dangerous hormone replacement therapies.

FOODS AND SUPPLEMENTS THAT CAN HELP BOTH SEXES

The only difference between male and female sex hormones is the amount of them. Both men and women have and need estrogen, progesterone, and testosterone to be healthy. Both are affected when levels fluctuate widely or become low.

DHEA

Supplementing with natural DHEA (dehydroepiandrosterone) can help relieve mild to moderate depression that starts in middle age. In the body, DHEA is a naturally-occurring hormone that is a precursor to testosterone and estrogen. Made by the adrenal glands, production dwindles starting in early adulthood. By age 70, DHEA production is reduced by about 20 percent.

In one study, published in a 2005 issue of *Archives of General Psychiatry,* treatment with DHEA resulted in a 50 percent reduction in depression symptoms in half the participants. Treatment with the supplement was associated with an increase in testosterone blood levels in both men and women.

Positive results were achieved in test subjects between 51 and 72 years of age with documented depression who were given DHEA at 30–90 mg/day by mouth for four weeks, with doses above 30 mg/day divided into two or three doses per day. One of the treatment-resistant patients received DHEA for six months. Her depression improved 48 to 72 percent.

Natural Progesterone Cream

Progesterone is a hormone present in the body of both males and females that regulates the entire endocrine system. This means that progesterone keeps all the other hormones in balance. When there is a deficiency in progesterone, the other hormones can become deficient.

Birth control pills contain synthetic progesterone and, after years of use, can cause PMS symptoms such as depression. It may take years more before the system fully stabilizes, if at all. A friend of mine had a reputation of being difficult. She lost jobs as well as her temper. She'd been on The Pill for 14 years. When she got pregnant, people around her noticed a big change in her mood. She was more patient, tolerant, and calm. Approximately six months after she gave birth, she was back to her old self. It turned out she wasn't producing enough progesterone, and it affected her attitude.

Next to making dietary changes, progesterone therapy is one of the most widely recommended treatments for PMS. In some women, progesterone therapy dramatically halts the awful depression, fatigue, and irritability commonly associated with PMS, but in others it has no effect—and often makes the symptoms worse. The reason, more and more doctors now believe, is the type of progesterone prescribed.

Joseph T. Martorano, M.D., director of the PMS Medical Group in New York City, says that synthetic progesterone, chemically formulated and administered, such as Provera, fails because it can't exactly duplicate the progesterone naturally produced in the body—and it can cause the body to produce less of it.

Other man-made hormones are called pregestagens. Once taken, they kill the body's appetite for its own natural progesterone. Over time the use of these drugs can make depression worse, not better.

The best form of progesterone is natural progesterone cream, plant-based, made from either soybeans or Mexican wild yam root (Dioscorea villosa). The plant steroids are processed through several fermentation steps to create a molecule exactly like that of human progesterone. Natural progesterone creams should contain at least 400 mg of natural progesterone per ounce. The cream is recommended for women and men.

If you are in California, I have to warn you

that you may find it difficult to purchase DHEA and progesterone cream as our rights to choose our own medical care are further eroded. Due to the connection between estrogen and breast cancer and despite a proven safety record, officials have proclaimed, through a piece of legislation called Proposition 65, that any natural hormone can be deemed hazardous, hence no company in California may sell it.

Natural progesterone cream is identical to that which is made by the human body. Natural progesterone is not listed as a potential carcinogen in any other state in the USA, it is routinely used in fertility clinics around the globe, and, most ironically, it actually helps counteract the carcinogenic effects of estrogen.

Synthetic hormone replacement therapies *aren't* banned, even though they contain *proven* cancer-causing synthetic estrogens and artificial progestins. Why? Because prescriptions given to consumers are conveniently excluded.

If you are in California, write your state representatives to stop this monopolistic sham, and join the National Health Federation (NHF), the largest and oldest health freedom organization in the world. Include your letters with your membership dues, and the NHF, through their lobbyist, will make sure they get to the right people and make the most difference.

The National Health Federation made it possible for you to buy supplements today and is responsible for your freedom to purchase, use, and continue to have them. Learn more at the National Health Federation website, www.thenhf.com. Or contact The National Health Federation, P.O. Box 688, Monrovia, California 91017, 626-357-2181.

Minerals

When zinc levels were examined in people with depression, they were found to be low. This essential mineral is necessary for the formation of testosterone, with the severest cases of depression associated with low levels. Zinc is also important for the formation of serotonin. Symptoms of a zinc deficiency include psychosis, schizophrenia, dementia, anorexia nervosa, and attention deficit disorder.

A 13-year-old girl who was anorexic was able to overcome her disorder through zinc supplementation. After two weeks of supplementation with zinc (initially 15 milligrams daily, then 50 mg three times daily), her appetite and mood began to improve. After four months of supplementation, she gained weight and her depression cleared. Ten months after she stopped taking zinc, she became anorexic again, which improved once the zinc was reintroduced.

For optimum benefit, minerals should be taken together. They occur this way in nature, and your body needs them in combination. Calcium is not effective on its own. It needs magnesium and potassium to build bones. Zinc is balanced in the body by copper. Without it, zinc cannot be absorbed.

Remember, you're not what you put into your mouth; you're what you absorb and digest and deliver to cells. A mineral tablet is only one to five percent absorbable. Since the process of digestion is a process of liquefaction, your body has to take a hard rock tablet and turn it into solution. This may not be possible due to a number of factors, such as inadequate stomach acid, food allergies, intestinal problems, and stress. When you are under stress, your stomach muscles tighten, further restricting digestion.

This is why it is so important that when you decide to supplement, you target minerals in solution. For many years I have used Maximum Living's MineralRich, which is a tasty liquid mineral supplement that provides all the minerals, including zinc and copper, your body needs.

Vitamin B6 (Pyridoxine)

Depression is a relatively common side effect of oral contraceptives. But studies have found that vitamin B6 can help overcome such hormone-related side effects. Symptoms associated with birth control pills are pessimism, dissatisfaction, crying, and tension. Out of 22 depressed women who took The Pill, half of them saw improvement after taking only two milligrams of B6 twice a day for two months. A typical vitamin B6 dose is 50 mg/day.

If you could choose a food or supplement that would be the healthiest and most beneficial of all, what would you look for? First, it would be as close to the way God made it as possible. Every nutrient would be derived from natural sources, not synthesized. Next, it would include all the vitamins, minerals, and natural herbs that are needed for optimum health.

The most beneficial vitamin and mineral supplement on the market today is Maximum Living's Vita-Sprout. It has all the nutrients discovered to be beneficial today, including freeze-dried sprouts, vegetables, and herbs. And to make sure the entire complex of B vitamins are digested and assimilated properly, it includes friendly-body bacteria acidophilus. Nothing could be more complete for your immune system team than this power-packed, God-given formula.

Protein and Fat

Protein helps increase testosterone levels, but choosing fatty protein will send you back five spaces. Saturated fat from meat and trans fats from processed meats are rich in aromatase, an enzyme that turns testosterone into various estrogens. While I'm on the subject of meat and hormones, I have largely given up meat after discovering the myriad of fat-enhancing hormones that are being fed to cows, pigs, and chickens. Nobody has been able to assure the meat-eating consumer that these hormones don't end up in our bodies in harmful amounts.

For meatless protein that is complete, combine whole grains with legumes (beans, peas, and lentils). Whole grains, particularly brown rice and oatmeal, are also good sources of protein and energy and are preferable to processed grain products, such as white rice or white flour.

Soy is a good protein source, and Maximum Living Nutrition Bites are an excellent way to supplement deliciously. It is packaged as chewy nuggets and comes in three flavors: chocolate, vanilla nut, and peanut butter. The soy protein in these tasty snacks contains many other vital nutrients, including fiber and amino acids. Because they are natural, they have tryptophan, a serotonin precursor.

Vital Vegetables

To boost your hormone health, eat more broccoli, cabbage, and Brussels sprouts. A recent study showed these veggies to be rich in indole-3-carbinol (I3C), a phytochemical known to turn "bad" estrogens (which shut down testosterone production) into good ones (which help restore its production).

Aim for two servings a day of the various cruciferous vegetables, which include broccoli, Brussels sprouts, cabbage, collards, cress, kale, kohlrabi, mustard greens, bok choy, radishes, turnip greens, and watercress. If you can't handle these, 300 mg of diindolylmethane (also called DIM or diindolin), which is derived from I3C, does much the same thing. DIM can be purchased at most vitamin stores and through Internet companies.

In the next chapter, I will show how chemicals in our food, water, and environment contribute to depression and fatigue, and what you can do to protect yourself.

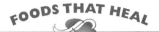
CHAPTER THREE

CHEMICAL FATIGUE

> *If life is a bowl of cherries,*
> *what am I doing in the pits?*
> —Erma Bombeck

MELANIE IS HOMELESS—driven from her home by chemicals. For over two years she has lived in a van, traveling from town to town in search of chemical-free air. As a child, she became sick from mercury amalgam fillings, chlorinated water, cortisone prescribed for rashes, and cleaning products. As an adolescent, she was depressed and nervous and had to quit school. As an adult, she endured trips to doctors and diagnoses of chronic fatigue, fibromyalgia, rapid heartbeat, sinus infection, and even menopause. It took three years to get a diagnosis of chemical sensitivity due to chemical overexposure. Drift from frequent aerial pesticide applications finally drove her from her home in search of clean living.

MULTIPLE CHEMICAL SENSITIVITY

Thirty percent of Americans suffer from multiple chemical sensitivity (MCS). Eighty percent of them are women. No longer rare, MCS sufferers experience symptoms that range from the mild (headaches, fatigue) to the severe (chest pains, depression, shortness of breath). Despite its growing frequency, however, MCS is rarely taken seriously. Conventional medicine does not know how to explain it, and doctors often proclaim its symptoms as psychogenic, or psychosomatic—originating in the patient's mind. This has left people, such as Melanie, in limbo. They are told they are crazy, or imagining their disease, or making it up, and they find themselves passed from physician to physician without answers or relief from their very real distress.

MCS is not new. People have been reporting its symptoms for the last 50 years, as our society has become more and more synthetic. Between 1940 and 1980, the production of synthetic organic chemicals increased from less than 10 billion pounds per year to more than 350 billion. In some ways, MCS is an allergy to modern life—a physical reaction to the common chemicals, ranging from detergents, pesticides, solvents, and perfumes to foods and pharmaceuticals, that permeate our everyday existence. Less than one percent of the 1,000 new chemicals added each year have been tested for toxicity.

Did you know that many of the ingredients in your perfume are the exact same ingredients found in gasoline? The scary thing is that the perfume industry is not regulated at all—they can put any number of chemicals in fragrance without

revealing what those chemicals are or how they affect humans.

Sodium lauryl sulfate, which is in many shampoos and skin care cleansers, is a known carcinogen and is added to shampoo to make it sudsy. Reported side effects include asthma, muscle aches, and fatigue. Symptoms of exposure can persist for more than two years and can be activated by common pollutants, such as automobile exhaust, perfumes, and passive smoking. It is amazing that a chemical that causes Multiple Chemical Sensitivity and cancer is allowed to be in our shampoo.

Propylene glycol, a chemical contained in antifreeze and brake fluid, associated with kidney problems, liver abnormalities, and skin problems, is a common ingredient in beauty creams, cleansers, and cosmetics.

Fortunately, there are skin care products available that don't contain this and other synthetic chemicals. I formulated the Eden Formulas skin care line without any synthetic chemicals at all. Every one of the Eden Formula products contain only natural ingredients.

THE IMMUNE CONNECTION

Chronic fatigue syndrome, fibromyalgia, and even post-traumatic stress disorder have symptoms so similar to MCS that researchers now theorize they may share a common cause.

Chemical intolerance is another name for

MCS. In one study, 60 percent of solvent-exposed workers reported having chemical intolerance. Up to half of patients with chronic fatigue syndrome and fibromyalgia, as well as a many Gulf War veterans, have chemical intolerance.

Names for this problem also include Gulf War syndrome, allergic toxemia, neurotoxicity, environmental allergy, 20th Century disease, sick building syndrome, ecologic illness, and toxic carpet syndrome.

One theory is that it results from an impaired immune system. It is like a barrel that continually fills with chemicals until it overflows and symptoms appear. Some also say that a single serious episode of infection, stress, or chemical exposure can cause the immune system to break down.

VITAMIN C FOR IMMUNE FUNCTION

Research has backed up this immune system theory. One study found that 55 patients between 28 and 65 years of age who had documented evidence of exposure to toxic chemicals also had low natural killer cell, T and B cell function.

It stands to reason that for anyone sensitive to chemicals, treatment would entail natural nutrients derived from God-given foods. The 55 patients were given 60 mg per kg of body weight of buffered vitamin C. (An 160-pound woman would be given four grams—4,000 milligrams.) Exactly 24 hours after the vitamin C was given, natural killer cell activity was increased up to tenfold in 78 percent of the patients. Patients who responded were advised to continue that dose on a daily basis. Vitamin C is also important to the metabolism of serotonin.

Vitamin C, or ascorbic acid, is the star player in your immune system. When levels are low, the body suffers for it. When the body responds adversely to chemicals, it uses up large amounts of vitamin C.

Because it isn't stored in or produced by the body, vitamin C must be taken regularly. In order to achieve a therapeutic healing effect, vitamin C must be continually retained in the body. And since the body excretes what it does not immediately need, high doses must be taken at regular intervals throughout the day.

The first thing you need to do is determine how much vitamin C you need to take to make your body well. The amount is determined by how much your body will absorb before it excretes it in the form of a small amount of diarrhea. This is called "bowel tolerance."

Begin with 5,000 milligrams. Two hours later take 1,000 milligrams. Continue taking 1,000 milligrams every hour—or 2,000 milligrams every two hours—and continue until you experience diarrhea or gas, then lower the amount to just below that.

You need not do this every day. You do this only to establish the amount you need to make your own body well. For most healthy people, the vitamin C dosage is three to six grams a day (3,000–6,000 milligrams). But when we are ill, our tolerance—and thus our body's need—may increase to 20 to 30 grams per day.

Vitamin C has been used to pull cadmium, lead, and nickel out of the body, as well as help the body overcome drug overdoses. Interestingly, long-term drug addicts take high doses of vitamin C with their drugs. Perhaps they know something we are just learning.

Always take vitamin C in a supplement formula that includes bioflavonoids. In nature, vitamin C and bioflavonoids go together, forming the most potent form of defense against illness and inflammation. To protect myself, I never travel without my Maximum Living Solu-C with green tea. It combines the health-giving bioflavonoids rutin, quercetin, and green tea with vitamin C to protect me against being ravaged by clouds of chemicals.

ENZYMES AND AMINO ACIDS TO OVERCOME CHEMICAL POISONING

Enzymes and amino acids keep poisons and synthetic chemicals from being absorbed and help pull them from the body.

To remove chemical poisons from your body take supplemental enzymes on an empty stomach so they are absorbed in the intestine and bloodstream. Once in the bloodstream, they are able to fight disease. When taken like this, enzymes mimic the benefits of enzyme-packed food, such as fresh fruits and vegetables, helping prevent the symptoms of chemical poisoning. Enzymes stimulate the body's own natural healing processes without causing the immune system to be suppressed (as occurs when cortisone is used to fight inflammation).

When you are exposed to chemicals, take Maximum Living's Multi-Enzyme formula. For detoxification and systemic relief, choose Maximum Living's "extended release" Enzyme-Ease.

There are approximately 22 amino acids that are components of protein. Eight of these cannot be manufactured by the body and must be supplied by food or supplementation. They are called free-form amino acids. Three of these are also antioxidants, further helping the body withstand the stresses of infection and illness. They are cysteine, glutathione, and methionine.

The amino acids cysteine and methionine help rid the body of toxins and poisons. A lack of cysteine is directly correlated with AIDS and other immune-deficiency ailments, and cysteine has been used to treat patients with HIV-1 infection.

Glutathione levels in the body are such a strong predictor of immune health that it is used as a measurement. Vitamin C and the mineral selenium, both antioxidants, increase levels of glutathione. Researchers at the National Institutes of Health found that the immune cells of AIDS patients are glutathione deficient.

Tryptophan, an amino acid found naturally in the body, is important to mental health, pain regulation, and sleep. Stress depletes it, and tryptophan is found to be deficient in people with depression and fibromyalgia. Not enough tryptophan and serotonin levels are low. European physicians prescribe tryptophan for insomnia, pain, stress. and depression. Tryptophan works most efficiently in the presence of plenty of vitamin B6. Women who take oral contraceptives need a minimum of 20 milligrams of vitamin B6 daily in order to absorb tryptophan.

Amino acids are like the slats of a barrel. You need the full set, and one is only as effective as the shortest slat. For full supplemental benefit, look for a formula that includes all the free-form amino acids, such as Maximum Living's amino acid formula, which is all natural; derived from a hypoallergenic whey source.

The same goes for the B vitamins. They must be taken together for optimum benefit. Again, turn to Maximum Living's Vita-Sprout. It includes the entire complex of B vitamins, including 30 milligrams of vitamin B6 and minerals such as selenium.

CHELATION NUTRIENTS—POWERFUL DETOXIFIERS

I hope Melanie—wherever she is today—reads this. It may allow her to come home.

Chelation therapy, controversial and condemned by convention for the treatment of heart and circulation problems, is the conventional therapy of choice in the case of lead or heavy metal poisoning. Chelation (key-lay-shun) comes from the Greek word *chele*, meaning to claw or bind. It is accomplished by giving the patient EDTA (ethylenediaminetetraacetic acid) intravenously. Chelation therapy is performed on an outpatient basis, is painless, and takes approximately 3-1/2 hours. For optimal results, physicians who use chelation therapy recommend 20–30 treatments given at an average rate of one to three per week.

In 1948, the U.S. Navy began using EDTA to safely and successfully treat lead poisoning. At the same time, EDTA was being used to remove calcium from pipes and boilers. EDTA is approved by the FDA for heavy metal toxicity.

For maximum benefit, EDTA therapy should be accompanied by a carefully tailored program of vitamin and nutritional supplements.

One physician I know treats lead poisoning with a combination of 30–40 grams of vitamin C intravenously, at frequent intervals, and less severe cases with oral doses of vitamin C and minerals in solution. One of his patients, a three-year-old boy who had been exposed to lead from the air and soil of a crowded trailer park near a busy freeway, was given five grams of vitamin C initially with minerals in solution, 400 IU of vitamin D, and a B complex formula that contained at least

25 mg of vitamin B6. The boy's symptoms—dark circles under the eyes, poor appetite, lethargy, sallow appearance—subsided in four to six months.

Electric battery factories are notorious for lead-polluted air. Researchers at the Brain Bio Center in Princeton, New Jersey did a study of 22 factory employees with lead poisoning. They were given 2,000 milligrams of vitamin C and 60 mg of zinc each day, and within 24 weeks their blood levels of lead plummeted by 26 percent.

EDTA is toxic in high doses and should not be used for children. They should, instead, be treated with high amounts of vitamin C to bowel tolerance.

THE QUESTION OF FOOD ADDITIVES

What about chemical food additives? Nobody knows for sure. According to Michael Jacobson, Ph.D., director of the Center for Science in the Public Interest in Washington, D.C., "Food additives are not normally tested for neurotoxicity or for how they interact with other food agents."

There are over 14,000 man-made chemicals added to our American food supply today. Included among these are antibiotics given to meat-producing animals, anti-foaming agents, foaming agents, bleaches, chemical sterilizing agents, coating materials, colorings, emulsifiers, flavorings, artificial smoke, modifiers, organic solvents, preservatives, sweeteners, synthetic dyes, and thickeners.

Add one more item to the list of to-dos: organically grown and additive-free foods. They are the best bet for your brain.

For more on boosting the immune system, read my booklet *Achieving Super Immunity.* In the meantime, for more on foods to eat and how diet influences mood, read on to the next chapter.

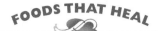

CHAPTER FOUR

DEPRESSION AND DIET

Volumes are written and spoken about the effect of the mind upon the body. Much of it is true. But I wish a little more was thought of the effect of the body on the mind.

—Florence Nightingale

KAREESHA JODHPURIA didn't know what to think when she woke up with double vision. She saw three eyes when she looked in the mirror, and she was dizzy. She shook her head, as though she could shake herself into balance. Her hands trembled violently as she picked up the phone and called her sister to take her to the hospital.

At the advice of a psychiatrist, Kareesha was taking lithium for depression. After much consultation and time, leaving Kareesha to wonder if she had a brain tumor, it was determined that the prescribed lithium dosage had been too high, and her psychiatrist suggested she try lowering it. Fed up with being a guinea pig and certain there was a better solution, Kareesha threw out her prescriptions and talked to a nutritionist. Tests determined Kareesha had a B-vitamin and fatty acid deficiency. She changed her diet—more fish and less meat; no coffee, sugar, hydrogenated oils, or salt—and noticed a marked improvement in her mood. She was never tempted to try lithium or antidepressants again.

A survey conducted by a British mental health group found that 80 percent of those who followed a diet low in sugar, caffeine, chocolate, and alcohol, and high in water, vegetables, fruit, and oil-rich fish reported improved mental health, with 26 percent citing major improvement.

What you eat and ingest has a far greater impact on your mental health than you realize. Food allergies, nutritional deficiencies, and natural stimulants, such as refined sugar, alcohol, simple carbohydrates, and caffeine, can mean the difference between a satisfying life and clinical depression.

CHEMICALS IN FOOD

In the last chapter I discussed chemicals in food. What's in that loaf of bread you just bought at the market? Have you read the label? It's crammed with synthetic chemicals designed to make the bread look appealing and stay soft on the grocer's shelf until you buy it. Many studies have shown children with behavioral disorders often have chemical sensitivities. All processed foods, whether bottled, bagged, canned, or packaged, have hidden dangers.

Monosodium glutamate (MSG) is only one of the identified dangers lurking in the plethora of chemicals contained in processed food. A very good friend of mine has migraines for days after ingesting MSG. Unfortunately, he eats out often and forgets to ask the waitress to "Hold the MSG."

Sulfites are preservatives found in many processed foods—and in most U.S. wines. They may preserve food, but sulfites deplete the body of thiamine, an essential nutrient that when deficient can cause depression. Many chemicals can also drain the body of essential nutrients, compounding the problem.

If there is any chance at all that you are chemically sensitive, stay away from processed foods. Some supermarkets are proclaiming their produce is free from pesticide residues. What they don't tell you is the food is often grown in chemically-fertilized or chemically-sterilized soil.

Carol Channing's friends joke that the musical-comedy star is almost as famous for her offstage eating habits as for her public performances. Channing has suffered for many years from an allergic reaction to chemicals used in food production and preparation. When on tour, she travels everywhere with special organic foods packed in silver *Tiffany* containers, and additional supplies are shipped to her by airmail—even if she's invited by the Queen of England to dinner at Buckingham Palace.

DETOXIFYING GARLIC

Have you heard of the Garlic Diet? You don't lose much weight, but from a distance your friends think you look thinner.

If the power is in the smell, then garlic is tops. It contains 33 sulfur compounds; 17 amino acids; germanium (good for controlling the effects of stress), selenium (mineral antioxidant), and a host of other important vitamins and minerals.

Garlic is rich in sulfur-containing compounds that cleanse and empower the immune system—both enhancing overall immune function and strengthening killer T-cells. Some of its sulfur compounds bind to heavy metals, such as lead and mercury, and neutralize them. Garlic also strengthens the liver, the organ most affected by chemicals.

The most therapeutic compound in garlic—allicin—is not released unless finely chopped, and then it diminishes over time and with cooking. Microwaving destroys allicin. Garlic is also extremely caustic. It can burn the skin and, internally, too much can damage the digestive tract. For these reasons, if you want the full medicinal benefit take supplemental garlic, which isolates and retains the most effective ingredients until you are ready to use it.

I highly recommend Maximum Living Garlic

Tabs. It contains the active compounds allicin and alliin as well as detoxifying glutathione and antioxidant vitamins A, C, and E.

FOOD ALLERGIES

Sensitivity to certain foods can also cause depression. I'm not talking about your neighbor crying when she runs out of chocolate, although there is a connection. I'm talking about hyperactivity and attention deficit disorder in kids, depression, headaches, mood swings, and even PMS. All are symptoms of food allergies.

Black circles under the eyes can indicate a food allergy, as can multiple horizontal wrinkles under the lower eyelid caused by allergic swelling.

The trouble with food allergies is what they do to your body, most importantly to your intestines. I knew a woman who had an allergy to gluten—called celiac disease. Before she was finally diagnosed, all the cilia in her intestine were destroyed. She wasn't able to assimilate nutrients and could only live through liquid supplementation. The B vitamins—vital to the nervous system—are absorbed in the intestines. If there is something wrong with the intestines, nutrients cannot be absorbed properly, especially the B vitamins.

B VITAMINS FOR MENTAL HEALTH

There are no other nutrients more important to mental health than the B vitamins. The B-complex vitamins provide the body with energy, metabolizing fats and protein, and are necessary for the normal functioning of the nervous system. They are the single most important factor for the health of the nerves.

Studies have shown that among those with intestinal problems, their blood levels of B vitamins are low. Irritable bowel syndrome (IBS) is a fancy term to describe a temporarily dysfunctional large intestine, caused by food allergies, stress, or too much fat in the diet.

In one study, 20 patients with IBS were compared to a control group of 20 without IBS. Remarkably, but not surprisingly, it was found that 18 out of 20 of the IBS patients had a history of mental illness during their lifetimes compared to only nine out of 20 in the control group. Half of the patients with IBS had regular panic attacks, and another half had social phobias. IBS patients commonly have problems with depression, sleeping problems, and substance abuse. The connection sticks. When questioned, most of the IBS patients said their intestinal problems occurred before their mental illness.

A vitamin B12 deficiency can produce psychosis, severe memory loss, impaired abstract thinking skills, mental confusion, delusions, hallucinations, and even brain and spinal cord degeneration (causing numbness). Low blood levels of the vitamin are found in one third of hospitalized psychiatric patients suffering from depression and dementia, according to a Denmark study.

Foods that serve as B12 boosters include liver, crab, herring, red snapper, flounder, salmon, lamb, Swiss cheese, eggs, haddock, cottage cheese, and swordfish.

Folic acid, a B vitamin found in leafy greens, prevents irritability and forgetfulness. In one case, 67 percent of patients admitted to a psychogeriatric ward were deficient in folate.

Foods high in folic acid are avocados, brown rice, wheat bran, soybeans, bean sprouts, artichokes, beets, cauliflower, and corn.

Vitamin B6, or pyridoxine, is the cofactor for enzymes that convert L-tryptophan to serotonin. Consequently, a vitamin B6 deficiency can result in depression. One person volunteered to eat a pyridoxine-free diet for 55 days. The resultant depression was alleviated soon after supplementation with B6 was begun. In one study, 21 percent of 101 depressed outpatients had low blood levels of the vitamin. In another study, four of seven depressed patients had a B6 deficiency.

Foods high in vitamin B6 include brewer's yeast, brown rice, whole wheat, royal jelly, soybeans, rye, lentils, sunflower seeds, hazelnuts, alfalfa, salmon, wheat germ, tuna, bran, walnuts, peas, and beans (legumes).

A vitamin B1, or thiamine, deficiency, called beriberi, is known to cause mental problems. Even a moderate thiamine deficiency can cause anxiety or neuroses. In one study, subjects deprived of thiamine complained of poor mental alertness, fatigue, and nervousness. Since psychiatrists are the least likely to inquire about diet, I have to wonder how many of their mental patients are being treated with drugs when they are simply thiamine-deficient. More on *that* later.

Stay away from the candy counter! A diet high in empty calories and junk foods has been linked to "neurotic behavior." In one study, 20 patients with a thiamine deficiency reported symptoms including aggressiveness and hostility. Of the 20, 12 reported a diet high in carbonated and other sweet beverages, candy, and typical snack foods. Blood tests indicated that all 20 had low thiamine levels. After the patients were given thiamine supplements, all 20 had marked improvement or lost their symptoms completely.

If you are anxious, depressed, or suffer from neuroses, consider the possibility that you have beriberi. In the meantime, target foods high in thiamine: brewer's yeast, wheat germ, rice bran, whole grains, beans, peas, and nuts.

Remember, the B vitamins must be taken together, so do the B complex shuffle with Maximum Living's Vita Sprout. The whole B complex family includes B1 (thiamine), B2 (riboflavin), B3 (niacin), B5 (pantothenic acid), B6 (pyridoxine), B12 (cobalamin), B15 (pangamic acid), biotin, choline, folic acid, inositol, and PABA (para-aminobenzoic acid). Each B vitamin has its own role in body function, centered on the nervous system. Since nerves bring messages to all the organs and stimulate glands to secrete their important biochemicals, the whole body communication system can break down with a B vitamin deficiency.

LOW BLOOD SUGAR

Another food-related cause of depression is hypoglycemia or low blood sugar. Glucose, or blood sugar, is the main energy source of the brain. When there is inadequate amounts, the brain—and your mood—suffers.

Low blood sugar is caused by not eating, or by eating what I call non-foods: white bread, white rice, most processed foods, and sugary snacks. I call white bread, sugar, and coffee stimulant foods because they quickly raise the blood sugar or stimulate the body, but just as quickly bring the body down, affecting the mood. Those used to having regular cups of coffee experience headaches and lethargy when coffee is not available.

Hypoglycemia raises cortisol levels. Cortisol is the body's major stress hormone. Its production is increased by all types of stress: mental/emotional, nutritional-chemical, physical, physiologic, and environmental. If you remember from the hormone chapter, high cortisol levels cause depression.

Depression is prevalent and often chronic among those with diabetes due to low blood sugar. Even if you are not diabetic, the same effect occurs when you eat foods that digest quickly—

called high glycemic food—because they cause the blood sugar to rise quickly, then fall.

Forgive me if I borrow from my booklet on diabetes, *Preventing and Conquering Diabetes*. This information is also valid for those with depression and fatigue.

People with diabetes learn to measure their blood sugar levels before, during, and after meals because what they eat is so important. They learn which foods keep their blood sugar stable and which can put them into a coma.

If you experience bouts of depression before or after meals, what you are eating could be the culprit.

The speed at which a food is able to increase a person's blood glucose levels is called the glycemic response. The glycemic response is influenced by many factors. Some factors may be the amount of food you eat (ideally small portions), how the food is processed (as little as possible), or the way the food is prepared. Pasta cooked "al dente" (firm) is absorbed more slowly than pasta that is overcooked.

The Glycemic Index is a ranking of foods based on their immediate effects on blood sugar levels. This index measures how much a person's blood glucose increases over a period of two or three hours after a meal. A food with a moderate Glycemic Index can be lowered by cooking or processing it less, and made even lower by eating small portions slowly. In order to keep blood sugar—and mood—stabilized, you should eat foods with a low Glycemic Index. Foods with a low number, by the way, also burn fat. Nothing wrong with that!

Where do you think bread ranks? The highest GI food most commonly found on the American dinner plate is white bread. It's in pizza and just about every fast food meal out there. The rank of white bread is 100.

The lowest foods are the ones closest to nature: raw and unrefined. For a short list of low glycemic foods, see my diabetes booklet. It would be impossible to list every food and its index rating, so if you have access to the Internet and want to know the rating of a specific food search, "glycemic apple," for example. This technique is widely used, and there is much information available.

NUTRITIONAL DEFICIENCIES

A deficiency of the mineral magnesium can cause numerous psychological changes, including depression. The symptoms of magnesium deficiency include poor attention, memory loss, fear, restlessness, insomnia, tics, cramps, and dizziness.

In a study of more than 200 patients with depression, 75 percent had white blood cell magnesium levels below normal. Intravenous magnesium not only helped their muscle pain but their depression also improved. Magnesium has also been used to treat premenstrual mood changes.

Dietary surveys have shown that many Americans don't get even the Recommended Dietary Allowance for magnesium. I'm not surprised since foods highest in magnesium are not found so readily at fast food joints or in the typical American diet. They are whole wheat, pumpkin seeds, millet, almonds, Brazil nuts, hazel nuts, dark-green vegetables, and molasses.

Choose foods with the proper proportions of calcium, magnesium, and potassium, since they work together. These are: wheat germ, sunflower seeds, soybeans, almonds, Brazil nuts, pistachios, and pecans. If you like trail mix, you're in luck. It's the best snack for a healthy nervous system.

Remember, for a multiple mineral supplement, instead of hard tablets, choose a formula in solution, especially if you think you have food sensitivities or digestive problems. MineralRich also contains brain-boosting vitamin B12.

GOOD FATS NEEDED

The above mentioned nuts and seeds contain more than just minerals. They also contain essential fatty acids—the good fats that lubricate the nervous system. Technically, they make up brain cell membrane receptors for serotonin. In any case, without them we are in trouble.

When you consider the kinds of foods our ancestors ate and compare them with what we typically eat today, you can see where modern diseases, syndromes, and afflictions come from. If

McDonald's was the last place you ate fish, consider yourself warned.

Over the last century, the American diet has contained less and less fish, nuts, and seeds—omega-6 and omega-3 fatty acids. We are supposed to be getting omega-6 fatty acids from vegetable oils. But how nutritious can they be in clear bottles that sit for months on supermarket shelves? Ultraviolet light and heat destroys nutrients in food, especially oils, and unless synthetic preservatives are added, they become rancid. I stay away from supermarket oils.

Walnuts and sunflower seeds contain high amounts of omega-6 fatty acids, and if you get your walnut and sunflower oils from organic growers at a farmers market, so will they.

But it is omega-3 fatty acid that seems to have the most benefit for alleviating depression. Dietary sources of omega-3 fatty acids include flax and fish.

Fish with the highest amounts of omega-3 are Atlantic mackerel, albacore tuna, Atlantic herring, Chinook salmon, lake trout, Atlantic salmon, and bluefin tuna. It is recommended that we eat fish two to three times a week.

When buying fish, avoid those that have been raised in hatcheries or farms. Fish raised on processed food, usually corn, lack essential fatty acids, which are found in the wild.

Studies have shown that higher national consumption of fish for a nation equals lower rates of depression versus countries consuming the least amount of fish. Higher fish consumption is also correlated with lower risk of postpartum depression and seasonal affective disorder. Researchers are seeing increasing rates of depression in regions of the world that are moving away from traditional omega-3-rich diets to typical Western foods.

If you really don't like fish or can't eat this much fish, supplement with Maximum Living flaxseed oil. The oil extracted from flaxseed is generously rich in omega-3 fatty acids and also contains naturally-occurring vitamin A, E, trace minerals, and amino acids—all important to good mental health.

HERBAL REMEDIES FOR SYMPTOMS

If you suffer from depression, please have your nutritional status tested to make sure you don't have B vitamin deficiencies. The success of alternative remedies for symptoms can still make us forget to identify the underlying cause.

Hypericum perforatum, also known as St. John's Wort, is a plant extract as effective as antidepressants with less severe side effects. Antidepressive medications often interfere with sleep, cognitive function, and memory while St. John's Wort may actually improve them. St. John's Wort is recommended for mild to moderate depression. Most St. John's Wort studies have used 300 milligrams taken three times a day.

Formulated from nature, Maximum Living's

Mood Assure is a comprehensive blend of St. John's Wort and the amino acid L-theanine, a component of green tea that encourages a relaxed state through its influence on the production of serotonin. Other ingredients include brainy B-vitamins, muscle-relaxing minerals calcium and magnesium, and hormone-helping zinc and copper.

Ginkgo biloba is one of the oldest living tree species, and its leaves are among the most extensively studied botanicals in use today. In Europe, it is among the best-selling herbal medications, and it ranks within the top five of all prescriptions written in France and Germany.

Ginkgo is used to treat circulatory disorders and enhance memory. It is especially helpful in increasing blood flow to the brain. Patients suffering from varying degrees of circulation problems who took ginkgo biloba extract also noticed an improvement in mood. One study showed reduced brain blood flow in depressed patients older than 50 when compared with those of the same age but not experiencing depression. This has prompted a surge of interest in ginkgo's use for depression in older people.

Maximum Living offers Ginkgo Biloba with DHA (docosahexaenoic acid). DHA is essential for the growth and development of the brain in infants, and it is required for the maintenance of normal brain function in adults. One of the reasons fish oil is so beneficial for depression is the fact that DHA is an active component of fatty fish (such as salmon, tuna, mackerel). Several large-scale studies have found a clear association between low blood levels of DHA and an increased risk of depression.

SUPPLEMENTAL TREATMENTS TO TRY

Another supplement worthy of consideration in the treatment of depression is S-Adenosyl-Methionine (SAM). When given as a supplement, SAM increases serotonin and has been found to be beneficial in treating depression.

Nicotinamide Adenine Dinucleotide, or NADH, is produced by the body. It is available in supplemental form and has been found in studies to alleviate depression. NADH increases energy in body cells and is a potent antioxidant.

Phosphatidylserine is found in the cell membranes of the brain and suppresses cortisol, the stress hormone mentioned before. It has been found to be helpful for elderly people experiencing depression.

SAD REASONS FOR DEPRESSION

In the next chapter I will cover other reasons for depression; possibilities you may not have thought of. Would you believe a yeast infection can cause depression? It's true! Not enough sunlight is also a culprit. Follow along while I explain all.

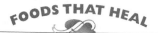

CHAPTER FIVE

OTHER REASONS FOR DEPRESSION

The term "clinical depression"
finds its way into too many
conversations these day.
One has a sense that a
catastrophe has occurred in the
psychic landscape.

—*Leonard Cohen*

THE NEXT TIME YOU ARE ON A TRAIN, in a theater, or in a crowd, look at the peoples' faces. I do, all the time. I look for people who need help; people whose skin tone, posture, and demeanor beg for relief and answers. Sometimes I approach, gently asking if there is anything I can do. I think maybe God talks to them, giving them a little nudge, whispering in their ear to trust me; because sometimes they listen and hear what I say.

I met Ruth Ann during an intermission of the Broadway hit *Dirty Rotten Scoundrels* in New York last year. She was 38, but she looked 50. Her arms were weak, and she felt clumsy. She was depressed and having memory problems. She slept all the time and had cut back her work schedule. What struck a chord with me was her admission that she had been suffering from yeast infections and had taken many antibiotics in the past, including tetracycline for acne. I explained to her what you'll learn as you read on. I hope it helped.

YEAST INFECTIONS PRODUCE CHEMICAL TOXINS

Again, we are back to the chemical toxicity issue, because it turns out that when the body is overwhelmed with yeast (a type of fungus), such as Candida albicans, it infects the body with poisons. Eventually the yeast will penetrate the intestinal lining, allowing toxins and food allergens to leak into the bloodstream. The more they enter the bloodstream, the weaker your immune system becomes and the more sick and depressed you feel.

Candida has been found to produce 79 distinct poisons, which the body must dispose of. As they move throughout the body, no organ system is immune to their effects, including the brain. These poisons include alcohol and acetaldehyde, making the patient feel intoxicated just as if they were drinking alcohol. When acetaldehyde reacts with the brain chemical dopamine, it can cause anxiety, depression, poor concentration, and wooziness. It is no surprise, then, that depression and chronic fatigue are two of the most common complaints of people suffering from yeast overload.

ANTIBIOTICS AND YEAST INFECTIONS

Antibiotics can cause depression. How? Because chronic use of antibiotics leads to Candida infections. Candida is also caused by a diet high in refined carbohydrates—high glycemic foods such as sugar and white bread—which are the fungus' favorite foods. They thrive on them.

Instead of white bread, take advantage of today's multi-grain offerings. I eat a whole, seven-grain bread every day. Whole grains contain fungus-fighting intestinal enzymes and essential B vitamins, and they digest slowly.

Normally, Candida isn't a problem because intestinal bacteria keep it under control. But when bacteria are killed by antibiotics, for example, the bad guys can proliferate while the good guys are still down for the count. Keep in mind that antibiotics are also in the food supply, because antibiotic supplements are given to animals as treatment for diseases and are used as food additives.

Stubborn resistance and a strong offensive are the best solutions to defeating the persistent Candida fungus. This means putting back the beneficial bacteria that was missing in the first place.

Normal vaginal bacteria is called Doderlein's bacillus. The closest thing obtainable is lactobacillus acidophilus, a beneficial bacteria found in supplements, yogurt, and other cultured food. Always check the date on the container, package, or bottle for freshness. Make sure the label says "live cultures."

In a study involving 30 women at the University of California, Davis, researchers reported that lactobacillus acidophilus inhibits Candida albicans. An article in *The Lancet* reported 20 women with Candida were cured with preparations containing lactobacillus acidophilus.

Found in supplemental formulas are the body's disease-killing good-guy bacteria, lactobacilli and bifidobacteria. They perform many valuable duties: reduce blood ammonia levels, lower cholesterol levels, regulate the immune system, produce vitamins, especially the B vitamin/folic acid group, restore normal intestinal flora during antibiotic therapy, as well as inhibit the growth of yeast.

In recent years there has been a growing awareness of the medical use of beneficial bacteria, termed "probiotics" (from the Greek, "for life"). Maximum Living has responded to this need with Probiotic Blend, a formula containing four strains of beneficial intestinal microflora bacteria specially made to help overcome systemic infections such as Candida.

Take Maximum Living's Garlic Tabs as well. Numerous studies have been conducted on the antifungal properties of garlic, and researchers have found it works on Candida. The *Journal of General Microbiology* reported on a study of garlic and its effect on Candida albicans. No matter how the researchers diluted it, the garlic was able to reduce the overgrowth.

LOW THYROID AND DEPRESSION

Sally, a potential Olympic contender, was doing very well in her trials. Her times were good, and her energy and stamina were optimal. She was moving further along in her goals to try out for the U.S. Olympic team. Suddenly her times were down, and fatigue set in. She was helpless and went to her doctor for help. He told her she was overtraining, that her body could not handle the work. He told her she would have to quit. All her life Sally had trusted her doctor. He had gotten her this far, and she would have to trust his judgment. She stopped training and let the trials go on without her. Months went by, and she didn't get any better. During a relaxation trip to Europe, she had a breakdown and ended up in a hospital in Germany. Doctors told her that when her tests showed she had abnormally high serum cholesterol levels—odd in an athlete—their suspicions proved true: she had primary hypothyroidism. This is what was causing her fatigue and depression.

Since that time, physicians who specialize in sports medicine are being cautioned about this possibility. In one study, female runners with a history of persistent fatigue and deteriorating running performances were evaluated. All of them were diagnosed as having primary hypothyroidism—their thyroid glands were not producing adequate amounts of thyroid hormone.

It's impossible to know many people with

chronic psychiatric symptoms are suffering from a completely organic, treatable thyroid problem. Doctors tell them to go home and get some rest, when what they need is to be diagnosed and treated.

The late Broda O. Barnes, an internationally recognized thyroid authority, stated that approximately 30 percent of patients treated for low thyroid function suffer slight to deep depression, fatigue, anxiety, irritability, mental sluggishness, and poor memory.

Researchers at the Department of Psychiatry, University of North Carolina, evaluated 16 patients with hypothyroidism and compared them to 15 control subjects with normal thyroid function. They found 56 percent of those with low thyroid function had depression compared to 20 percent with normal thyroid function.

After reviewing numerous studies and reports on the role of the thyroid in mood disorders, Dr. Junichi Nomura, MIE University School of Medicine in Japan, believes that physicians dealing with depressed patients, especially the elderly or women with PMS, should have their thyroid functions tested. He also found that large amounts of thyroid hormones may be therapeutic for the treatment of depression.

Thyroid hormones are made from iodine and the amino acid tyrosine. Make sure your thyroid gland has enough iodine so it can function properly. A deficiency of iodine results in the development of a goiter, an enlarged thyroid gland. Take Maximum Living's amino acid formula for tyrosine.

Barnes stated that first generation hypothyroids can correct their condition by including iodine in the diet. MineralRich has iodine, as does kelp. Hypothyroids of the second generation or beyond can overcome depression and many other symptoms of low thyroid function by taking natural desiccated thyroid. In my experience, a good natural thyroid hormone is Armor Thyroid. It can be obtained inexpensively by contacting Dr. Salvadore Vargas at 1-888-396-3130.

Dr. Barnes' best contribution toward public awareness of thyroid problems was probably the Barnes Basal Temperature Test, a simple test that can be done by anyone in the privacy of their own home. Since your body temperature reflects your metabolic rate, which is largely determined by hormones secreted by the thyroid gland, the state of the gland can be determined by taking your temperature. All that is needed is a thermometer.

- Shake down the thermometer to below 95°F and place it by your bed before going to bed at night.
- Upon awakening, before getting out of bed, place the thermometer in your armpit for a full ten minutes, making as little movement as possible.
- After ten minutes, read and record the temperature and the date.

- Record the temperature for at least three mornings, preferably at the same time each day. Menstruating women should perform the test on the second, third, and fourth days of menstruation.

Your basal body temperature should be between 97.6°F and 98.2°F. Anything lower can indicate hypothyroidism; anything higher can indicate hyperthyroidism.

Certain nutrients are necessary for a healthy thyroid. Zinc, vitamin A, and vitamin E function together to manufacture thyroid hormone. A deficiency of any of these results in lower levels of active thyroid being produced. There may be a correlation between the low zinc levels common in the elderly and the high incidence of hypothyroidism. The B vitamins riboflavin (B2), niacin (B3), and pyridoxine (B6), and vitamin C are also necessary for normal thyroid hormone manufacture.

VIRAL CAUSES OF FATIGUE AND DEPRESSION

There are at least two viruses known to cause fatigue and depression in humans: the Borna virus and the Epstein Barr virus.

Infectious mononucleosis, termed the "kissing disease," was the first illness recognized as causing chronic fatigue. In the mid 1980s, as the AIDS epidemic spurred extensive research into viruses, more became known about the mononucleosis syndrome. Mononucleosis became Chronic Epstein-

Barr Virus (CEBV). A March 1988 report by a Centers for Disease Control (CDC) working group renamed it Chronic Fatigue Syndrome.

The Borna virus may be blamed for behavioral problems such as depression, schizophrenia, and bipolar disorder. As I mentioned in the first chapter, the Borna virus was first identified in horses. It is also found in many other animals but only recently in human psychiatric patients. Studies are showing there may be a direct correlation between mental illness and this virus. When patients were treated with antiviral medicines, they experienced rapid remission of their mental symptoms.

As many as 15 percent of psychiatric patients are infected with Borna, while no more than two percent of people in the normal population are infected. One U.S. clinician found nine of 17 schizophrenics and two of five bipolar patients to be Borna positive while none of his healthy controls tested positive.

NATURAL ANTIVIRALS

Who needs pharmaceuticals with their horrible side effects when you can treat viruses safely and naturally? Viruses, including the Borna and Epstein Barr, are treatable with nutritional supplementation.

Of them all, vitamin C with bioflavonoids is perhaps the best known antiviral. It is well established that vitamin C is vitally important to healthy white blood cells.

If you didn't believe it before, pay attention to this! Since 1971, 21 placebo-controlled studies have been done evaluating vitamin C's effect at a dose of 1 to 4 grams per day on the common cold virus. In every one of these 21 studies, vitamin C reduced the duration and severity of symptoms of the common cold by an average 23 percent.

The body uses vitamin C to fight infection, and when stores are low, the body suffers for it. Six grams (6,000 milligrams) a day of vitamin C during a cold or flu can maximize the body's battle. The diet of our ancestors contained 0.4 to 2 grams (400–2,000 mgs) of vitamin C per day. To establish your own personal dosage, take vitamin C to bowel tolerance.

For the best quality vitamin C, supplement with Maximum Living's Solu-C product, which contains immune-boosting bioflavonoids.

Over 50 years ago, scientists first discovered vitamin A's value in treating and preventing flu viruses. In 1942, Italian physician Di Salvatore Princi published his study results that showed mice had more resistance to an influenza virus if they were given vitamin A.

Zinc also possesses direct antiviral activity. In a double-blind clinical trial, zinc gluconate lozenges significantly reduced the average duration of common colds by seven days. These lozenges can be purchased at vitamin and health food stores.

Echinacea is a natural herbal antibiotic that was one of the primary healing nutrients in the nineteenth century. Historically, the herb has been used to fight tuberculosis, diphtheria, malaria, sepsis, meningitis, gangrene, boils, carbuncles, and abscesses.

Goldenseal is a native American medicinal plant introduced to early settlers by Cherokee Indians who used it as a wash for skin diseases, wounds, and for sore, inflamed eyes. Its roots are bright yellow, thus the name. Goldenseal root has acquired a considerable reputation as a natural antibiotic and as a remedy for various gastric and genitourinary disorders.

Andrographis paniculata (AP), also known commonly as "King of Bitters," is a member of the plant family Acanthaceae and has been used for centuries in Asia to treat a variety of chronic and infectious diseases. In traditional Chinese medicine (TCM), andrographis is used to dispel toxins from the body. In Scandinavian countries, it is commonly used to prevent and treat common colds.

The herbs mentioned above should be used only for short periods. Long-term use can alter the body's chemistry in such a way as to limit their immune beneficial effects. Andrographis paniculata should not be used by women who are pregnant, breastfeeding, or anyone trying to get pregnant.

These antiviral herbs are contained in Maximum Living's m-u Boost immune support product. I highly recommend it as a first course of treatment when chronic fatigue or depression gets you down.

SEASONAL AFFECTIVE DISORDER—SAD

So much for the theory of global warming! As we wait out the unseasonably rainy, cold days in anticipation of summer, something happens to us. We're tired, depressed, antisocial, and apathetic. We have trouble sleeping, and we eat like there's no tomorrow. Probably the biggest problem with this disorder is, knowing it will pass, we don't do anything about it. Life's too short, and the answer is simple.

An old Italian proverb explains: "When the sun does not enter, the doctor does." Recent discoveries of light's effect on hormone production have led to a term for these winter blues: seasonal affective disorder, appropriately, S.A.D. Approximately 11 million people in the United States, or six percent of the population, are afflicted by seasonal affective disorder.

Researchers discovered that the light-sensitive pineal, a tiny pine cone-shaped gland in the brain, plays a major role in determining behavior. Light travels via the pineal from the retina to the hypothalamus, a part of the brain believed to be involved in the running of our biological clock.

The modern use of light as a treatment for depression arose in the early 1980s from the investigations of sleep disturbances in seasonal and non-seasonal mood disorders. Alfred J, Lewy, M.D., Ph.D., then of the National Institute of Mental Health, published a study of normal human subjects showing that intense light can suppress nocturnal melatonin release. Melatonin is the hormone responsible for reproductive cycles and sleep, and because it can be measured in the blood, it has become a marker for the study of light's effect on behavior. Too little light convinces the body that it is time to sleep and inappropriately produces melatonin, which causes a depressed mood.

Preliminary SAD studies were conducted over several winters in the mid '80s at the National Institute of Mental Health. Participants had their day extended with bright light for three hours both at dawn and at dusk. The intensity of the light was five to ten times brighter than ordinary indoor light. Thirty out of the 34 participants showed significant improvement in mood and behavior within four days.

In one study, researchers subjected 54 people diagnosed with SAD to a cool-light, 2,500 lux fluorescent light for two weeks from 6 to 8 a.m. Following the therapy, the patients reported being able to sleep better and were not as depressed or apathetic.

Light therapy has been helpful among those who experience panic attacks during the winter months. One patient responded to a 2,500 lux light for five consecutive days from 5:30 to 7:30 a.m.

Previous light treatment entailed at least two hours of daily exposure to 2,500 lux light. More recent studies have shown that 10,000-lux light boxes (approximately 80 times brighter than the usual indoor lighting) require only 30 minutes of daily exposure to produce similar response rates. This treatment is more commonly used today.

THE DANGERS OF ANTIDEPRESSANTS

After decades of doctors prescribing antidepressants without care or cause, scientific and anecdotal evidence has forced the FDA to issue strong warnings against their use. In the next chapter I will cover which drugs are the most deadly, what to look for, and exactly what are their dangers and risks.

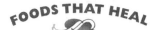

CHAPTER SIX

ANTIDEPRESSANTS AND THEIR DANGERS

> *Drugs are not always necessary,*
> *but belief in recovery always is.*
>
> —Norman Cousins

IN JANUARY 2006, four-time All-Star baseball pitcher Jeff Reardon, known as "The Terminator" and hero of the Minnesota Twins 1987 World Series team, blamed antidepressants after his arrest for a bizarre jewelry store robbery. Instead of walking out with valuable jewelry, he left with $170 in a bag. Reardon was so aghast by his own actions, he turned himself in to a security guard on the way out of the mall, explaining to the surprised guard, "I completely lost my mind." Later he told the police, "I flipped on my medications."

Was this just another contrived defense to get a troubled former athlete off the hook? Probably not. Having made over 11 million dollars over his career, why would he do it? Unfortunately, medical experts see this type of behavior over and over in patients who are using antidepressants. In

Reardon's case, following the death of his son by an overdose two years earlier, he stated that he had been taking five antidepressants compounded by a follow-up prescription after an angioplasty procedure a few days before the incident.

It's a simple fact that some people suffer anti-depressant-induced manic reactions that lead to actions that are totally out of character for them. And those actions are often far more dangerous and tragic than Reardon's.

TODAY'S ANTIDEPRESSANTS

The evidence against the use of pharmaceutical antidepressants is overwhelming and has been evident for over ten years. Yet they stay on the market and continue to be prescribed.

In 1991, 16,899 cases of adverse reactions from the use of Prozac were reported, with over 100 lawsuits filed against Eli Lilly, the manufacturer of the drug.

In September 1991, the FDA called a special hearing during the 34th meeting of the psychopharmacological drug advisory committee. A panel of "experts" were asked to hear testimony and then vote on the future of Prozac. Witnesses appeared before the panel and gave graphic accounts of sons and daughters who had taken their lives after ingesting the drug, of mothers fatally shooting themselves in front of their children, of lives destroyed or nearly destroyed; all pleading that Prozac be removed from the market.

The hearing came and went without any action by the FDA regarding the use of Prozac or other antidepressant drugs.

In 2002, doctors wrote nearly 11 million prescriptions for antidepressants to teenagers and children.

In 2003, children and adolescents made up about eight percent of patients prescribed antidepressant drugs in the U.S., constituting over ten million prescriptions dispensed for patients younger than 18 years. These drugs included Prozac, Paxil, Zoloft, Wellbutrin, and Celexa.

RECENT ACTION

In September 2004, FDA researchers analyzed 24 clinical trials involving 4,582 pediatric patients taking antidepressant medications for depression, anxiety, or other psychiatric disorders. FDA investigators concluded that patients taking antidepressants were *twice as likely* as patients taking placebo (fake) pills to experience suicidal thoughts or attempt suicide.

A month later, the FDA issued a Public Health Advisory to warn the public about the increased risk of suicidal thoughts and behavior in children and adolescents being treated with antidepressant medications. The FDA called for the labels of all antidepressants to have a "black box" warning about this risk. The new warning does not recommend they not be used for children and adolescents.

The FDA black box decision came some ten months after regulators in England declared that most antidepressants are not suitable for children under 18.

In February 2005, a study of data from 702 controlled clinical trials involving 87,650 *adult* patients found that those taking antidepressant drugs were *twice as likely* to attempt suicide as those receiving a placebo dummy pill or other treatments.

Soon after, a warning was issued by the FDA that prenatal exposure to antidepressants is linked to birth defects.

On June 30, 2005, the FDA issued a Public Health Advisory release entitled, "Suicidality in Adults Being Treated with Antidepressant Medications." The advisory states: "Several recent scientific publications suggest the possibility of an increased risk for suicidal behavior in adults who are being treated with antidepressant medications" and warns: "Adults being treated with antidepressant medications, particularly those being treated for depression, should be watched closely for worsening of depression and for increased suicidal thinking or behavior."

What else do you need to know about antidepressants?

Antidepressants may make people more depressed in the long term. Called the "oppositional model of drug tolerance," long-term drug treatment may cause the brain to react to counter the drugs' effects, leading to reduced effectiveness. When a drug is discontinued, the brain's oppositional process may continue, leaving an individual at high risk for a relapse.

Antidepressants can also lead to mental illness. A physician friend told me about a 35-year-old woman who took Prozac for only three days before she went from having mild depression with no suicidal tendencies to becoming acutely psychotic.

Any psychiatrist will tell you that excessive doses of antidepressants can cause brain dysfunction. This was commonly seen with early antidepressants such as Elavil and Tofranil. But the newer drugs, such as SSRIs (selective serotonin reuptake inhibitors), can also have severe side effects. They have been known to cause severe agitation or restlessness and a loss of impulse control. SSRIs are Prozac (fluoxetine), Cipramil (citalopram), Aropax (paroxetine), and Zoloft (sertraline).

Antidepressants can also trigger manic behavior in people whose depression is part of a manic-depressive syndrome, which often gets overlooked when people are given SSRIs. Dr. Ronald Pies, professor of psychiatry at Tufts University, wrote that "Some of these individuals may have serious adverse reactions to antidepressants, including irritability, aggression, and mania."

Sounds like Jeff Reardon, doesn't it?

HEALING THE SPIRIT

If you are reading this because you are newly

diagnosed with depression and are concerned about antidepressants, good for you. I have given you many alternatives to try. If you are reading this because you have been diagnosed with depression, have been given antidepressants, and want to try something else, please be warned that antidepressants combined with other brain chemical-altering substances—even safe natural herbals such as St. John's Wort—can cause problems.

Depression is little different than a broken leg. It requires interven tion and time to heal. The difference between the two is how people view it and the effect, as a result, this has on you. When body imbalances affect behavior, you may have to deal with not only the problem itself, but the disapproval and ignorance of others. This alone is depressing. So while you heal your body, the final chapter in this booklet will give you recipes to heal your spiritual, mental, and inner self, including the most potent stress-reducer of all, the one that has sustained and nourished me in times of challenges: a faith in God.

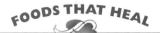

CHAPTER SEVEN

STRENGTHENING THE SPIRIT

Health is a state of complete physical, mental, and social well-being, and not merely the absence of disease or infirmity.

—*World Health Organization, 1948*

IN 1992, Peter was an introverted freshman at a high school dedicated to math, science, and the arts. That fall the school got connected with the Internet, which he attacked like a shark. With his math skills and passion for video games, he soon started programming and was able to hack into the school's computer system and change his grades, which nearly got him kicked out of school. Straight out of high school, his computer programming skills were so high that he was able get a job with an insurance company that allowed him to work at home.

After ten years of near total isolation, Peter is twenty-seven years old and spends most of his time in a small dark upstairs room in his rundown house whose doormat says "Go Away!" His neighbors consider him a recluse who's too paranoid to leave his house, although he does sneak out to the grocery stores in the middle of the night. What appeared to be a potentially brilliant career has gone nowhere. With a penchant for wordplay and constant television watching and other obsessions, the two constant factors in his life have been depression and aloneness. Peter is fortunate that his current addiction for guzzling rum will land him in chemical treatment program where he will rediscover the meaning and power of friendship and family.

ISOLATION IS TOXIC

Until now I have emphasized the physiology of depression and fatigue. The physical reasons need to be identified and resolved, but so too must the spiritual or mental needs be met in order to recover.

One point upon which everyone can agree: even among the most physically fit, isolation is toxic. Never assume you can get by without the support of people. The smartest thing you can do when troubled is seek out the support and help of others.

Reach out and form bonds, get involved with people, even on the most superficial level. You need not pour your heart out to everyone you meet in order to gain strength from their presence. Merely being in touch with the world and the people in it will lift your spirits.

Take a walk and observe others. See the children and how they delight in little things. See the animals and their comical peculiarities. Notice the happiness in others, and the beauty in nature. Marvel at man's accomplishments—architecture, literature, and technology. Make a strong concerted effort to see the positive in what's around you, and you'll be surprised at how much positive you see in yourself.

Look in the newspaper for club or organization meetings. Most of the time attendance does not require a commitment. You can enjoy the luxury of listening to others and appreciate their levels of involvement without having to invest your own. You may even learn something.

Give yourself a break. Rather than forcing yourself through a workday or workweek, laboring under your depression, take vacation or sick time. Let go of the burdens and concentrate on getting yourself well and making yourself happy again. Do what it takes to feel better.

GET OUT THERE

Social activities can bring you close to healthy people, many of whom are caring and who will help you recover without even knowing the extent of your problems. Church is the most ideal source of healthy activities. A wholesome environment is a Christian non-denominational church where the congregation is literally embraced in a spirit of fellowship and Christ-love.

This is backed by scientific study. In a survey of men and women 65 years or older, psychologists at the University of California, Los Angeles, found that elderly men reporting the recent death of a relative experienced markedly more depression than elderly women, and men who did not belong to a church or temple were more depressed by their loss than were men who had affiliation with a church or temple. The reasons for the gender gap in bereavement remain unclear, but one theory is that women have more social ties that help ease distress when a relative dies.

Another option for social outreach is a community college or community classes that offer stimulating courses and a positive atmosphere. Consider something you've always wanted to do or learn. Find a class and join.

The giving of oneself through volunteer work affords personal fulfillment, satisfaction, and acceptance. Service clubs—Scouts, PTA, Rotary, Kiwanis, Lions—are good bets for betterment and fulfillment. Get involved in local politics or community projects. Business and professional organizations can also prove helpful to recovery.

GET LESS SLEEP AND MORE EXERCISE

Have you noticed you feel more tired after getting more sleep? Depression is aggravated by too much sleep, seclusion, and stimulation avoidance. Seclusion from people, stimulation, and life in general deepens depression. A depressed person should do just the opposite: avoid seclusion, sleep less, and get exercise.

Most adults need about six to eight hours of sleep a night. Ironically, some people try to get too much, thinking more is better, and end up waking and tossing so much that their sleep isn't restful.

Dr. Michael J. Therapy, director of the Sleep/ Wake Disorders Center at Montefiore Medical Center in New York City, suggests a test to determine your optimum sleep pattern. To determine your sleep quota, go to bed at your usual time for one week. The second week, move your bedtime one hour later; the third week switch to one hour before your regular bedtime. The week in which it takes you five to 30 minutes to fall asleep and you wake up refreshed, and eventually without an alarm, is the one closest to your personal sleep quota.

Exercise is a vital part of a successful treatment program for depression. It tones and conditions the body and stimulates blood circulation in the brain. Work toward 30 to 60 minutes of moderate exercise daily. Brisk walking, swimming, and bicycling are excellent sustained activities. Start slowly and build up.

Exercise is any physical activity that is more than what you've done on a typical day. If you have been confined to your bed, or if you spend most of your day in front of the TV or on the computer because of your depression, then 15 minutes performing deep breathing exercises can be defined as "exercise." Later, when you feel better, your exercise level can progress to a 15-minute walk, then to a group aerobics class, swimming, or whatever exercise you choose.

At Purdue University, psychologists D. D. Lobstein and A. H. Ismail found that middle-aged professors who got exercise were much less depressed than the most sedentary of their colleagues.

Psychiatrists at the University of Wisconsin assigned 24 clinic patients with moderate depression to either an exercise program or one of two widely used forms of treatment. In the two standard treatment groups, therapists met with the patients once a week. In the exercise group, patients went jogging with a trainer three times a week for 45 to 60 minutes at a time. After 12 weeks, about three-quarters of the patients in each of the three treatment groups had gotten over their depression. But one year later, the people who had been treated with running therapy were still running on their own and were free of depression, while half of those who received psychotherapy had returned for treatment.

HAVE FAITH

The most convincing book I have read on the subject of faith-benefiting health is one I recommend with great joy and positive expectations. It is by Dr. Lester Sumrall and is entitled *Faith Can Change Your World*. It is available from Sumrall

Publishing, P.O. Box 12, South Bend IN 46624;
1-888-584-4847.

> *And we know that all things*
> *work together for good*
> *to them that love God,*
> *to them who are the called*
> *according to His purpose.*

—ROMANS 8:28

Also in this Series

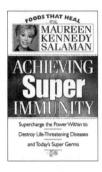

#610 / $7.95

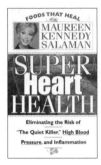

#625 / $7.95

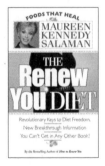

#620 / $7.95

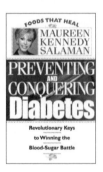

#630 / $7.95